Distribution, publication, and copying in any form are prohibited and subject to damages.

TEN HYPNOSES

Copying, publishing, and sharing with third parties are only permitted with the written consent of the author. Please observe the notes on copyright and usage.

Distribution, publication, and copying in any form are prohibited and subject to damages.

Copying, publishing, and sharing with third parties are only permitted with the written consent of the author. Please observe the notes on copyright and usage.

Ingo Michael Simon

TEN HYPNOSES

39
HEART ANXIETY NEUROSIS

Distribution, publication, and copying in any form are prohibited and subject to damages.

© 2024 Ingo Michael Simon
All rights reserved.
Independently published
www.ingosimon.com

Important Notes for Urgent Attention:

The contents of this book are based on the practical experiences of the author with hypnosis applications and psychotherapy in a trance state. Although the author has strived for the utmost care, errors or misunderstandings in the presentation cannot be completely excluded. Therapeutic work with people and the application of hypnosis are solely the responsibility of the hypnotist. It cannot be ruled out that parts of this book may be misunderstood or that the application of a presented procedure may cause an undesirable reaction in the client. The author also assumes no co-responsibility if work with a client is carried out with reference to the statements in this book.

The Author:

Ingo Michael Simon studied psychology and education and is a hypnotherapist with practices in southwestern Germany and Switzerland. With the help of hypnosis-supported psychotherapy, he primarily treats people with persistent psychological conditions. His practice focuses on anxiety disorders, pathological compulsions, and psychosomatic illnesses. His therapeutic offerings mainly include classical and modern hypnosis applications and the dreamland therapy he developed himself.

Copying, publishing, and sharing with third parties are only permitted with the written consent of the author. Please observe the notes on copyright and usage.

Distribution, publication, and copying in any form are prohibited and subject to damages.

INTRODUCTION — 6

COPYRIGHT AND USAGE — 8

HYPNOSIS 1 — 10

HYPNOSIS 2 — 15

HYPNOSIS 3 — 20

HYPNOSIS 4 — 25

HYPNOSIS 5 — 30

HYPNOSIS 6 — 35

HYPNOSIS 7 — 40

HYPNOSIS 8 — 45

HYPNOSIS 9 — 51

HYPNOSIS 10 — 57

ALL TITLES IN THE SERIES — 62

Copying, publishing, and sharing with third parties are only permitted with the written consent of the author. Please observe the notes on copyright and usage.

Introduction

The series "Ten Hypnoses" is very well known in Germany, Austria, and Switzerland as a collection of texts for therapeutic work and is used by numerous psychotherapeutic practices, doctors, therapists, coaches, and other helping professionals. I am pleased to now be able to offer these texts in other countries as well.

Most therapists have their own methods for inducing and deepening trance as well as for exiting trance. Therefore, I have focused on the main part of the hypnosis. The texts in this book can be integrated as the main part into any hypnosis process. The texts in this collection use various hypnosis techniques. I will not explain these in detail, as I assume that users have the appropriate training. It is also not necessary to understand the exact structure or functioning of the different parts. The texts can simply be read aloud, and they will have their effect.

Decide for yourself which text best suits your client or patient at any given time. You can also combine passages from different texts. It is not about using all ten hypnoses in sequence. It is a selection of possibilities.

I want to emphasize that books cannot replace therapy. Psychotherapy or other therapeutic treatments involve much more. A careful diagnosis is the necessary basis for deciding on the use of methods, including whether hypnosis or one of my texts should be used. Even in this case, preparatory discussions, follow-up discussions during the session, and of course, a therapeutic concept for the sequence of sessions and the content approaches are essential parts of therapy. This cannot and should not be achieved with a collection of texts.

In any case, I wish you much success in your work and I am pleased if my text templates can contribute in a small way.

Ingo Michael Simon

Copyright and Usage

Copying, publishing, and sharing with third parties is prohibited and only permitted with the written consent of the author. Please observe the following copyright and usage guidelines.

This work has been carefully crafted and created to the best of the author's knowledge and personal experience. It comprises text templates and application guidelines for professional hypnosis sessions. The author is a licensed psychotherapist with extensive experience in psychotherapy, coaching, and personal training using hypnotic techniques and methods. Nevertheless, the author and the publisher assume no liability for the accuracy of information, instructions, and advice, nor for any typographical errors. The author and publisher accept no responsibility or liability for the application of these texts and recommendations with clients or patients, nor for any potential consequences or unexpected reactions. It is expressly noted that the application of therapeutic and advisory techniques and formulations lies solely and entirely within the responsibility of the practitioner. This also applies to adherence to the boundaries of legally regulated medical and therapeutic practices. The fact that a book containing action proposals is freely available for sale does not imply that its application with clients or patients is permitted for everyone.

Hypnosis 1

You want to let go of fear today ... ... but you want even more ... ... You want to feel that your heart is healthy again ... ... because deep down, you know your heart is truly healthy ... ... Your mind knows it too ... ... Your heart is healthy ... ... Your heart is really healthy ... ... You're here today because you want to feel it too ... ... because you want to feel your heart beating normally again ... ... sometimes a little faster when you're excited or have been walking briskly ... ... But your heart always beats in a way that's right for your body ... ... You have this goal, to feel that again ... ... to always feel that everything is okay with your heart ... ... even when you think it's beating a bit faster ... ... Today, you're setting yourself up to maintain clarity and calm ... ... It's amazing how quickly you can do that ... ... really amazing how quickly you can adjust to the health of your heart ...

Our thoughts control our perception ... ... Thoughts can lead us to feel fear that isn't really there ... ... but they can also help us shift into a different feeling ... ... to return to our natural state of being ... ... So a good thought can help you ... ... a thought against fear ... ... a calming thought ... ... a thought for your healthy heart ... ... Thoughts are like beliefs ... ... The more we think them, the more solid they become ... ... and when that thought aligns with our deep inner feeling, it becomes a reality even faster ... ... and deep down, you know that your heart is completely healthy ... ... So you think ... ... I know my heart is healthy, and that's why I remain calm ... ... This one thought helps you stay calm and trust in the healthy function of your heart ... ... I know my heart is healthy, and that's why I remain calm ... ... This is your most important thought ... ... the thought of your health and your healthy heart ...

Your body awareness is particularly important when it comes to such a vital organ as the heart ... ... especially now ... ... the feeling in this very moment ... ... Right now, your body feels good ... ... You are inwardly calm and can become even calmer ... ... You feel at ease ... ... Your heart beats steadily and evenly ... ... Your heart is healthy ... ... Your heart beats calmly and rhythmically ... ... Your heart is very healthy ... ... You feel it now ... ... Right now, you feel the health of your heart clearly ... ... It beats steadily and calmly ... ... Even if you focus completely on your heart, you feel that it beats evenly and calmly because it is truly healthy ... ... Your body can relearn to signal this healthy state to you ... ... especially when you think your heart rate might be speeding up ... ... From now on, your body will help you stay calm ... ...

Fear is a feeling ... ... Calm is also a feeling ... ... Calm and composure ... ... Both cannot exist at the same time ... ... For example, right now you feel calm and relaxed ... ... So, you cannot feel fear ... ... So now, you focus all your mindfulness and attention on the feeling of calm within you ... ... The feeling of calm grows bigger and deeper ... ... The calm becomes stronger and deeper ... ... Each moment of conscious calm and relaxation dissolves thoughts of fear ... ... Each moment of conscious calm and relaxation builds new self-confidence ... ... new trust in your healthy heart ... ... because that is what you truly have ... ... a healthy heart ... ... You feel good ... ... really good ... ... Your heart beats steadily and evenly ... ... This calm feeling is pleasant and it stays with you all day ... ... Every day, you can experience this feeling anew ... ... the feeling of calm ... ... the feeling of health ... ... the feeling of a healthy heart ...

You are setting yourself up to do something that will always make it very easy to let go of troubling thoughts of fear and quickly return to inner calm ... ... You're already succeeding today ... ... You let go of fear for your heart, fear of heart disease, simply by not judging the fear anymore ... ... You feel it briefly and immediately move into your new helpful thought and fully immerse yourself in it ... ... I know my heart is healthy, and that's why I remain calm ... ... Your new thought then fills you completely and the fear fades away ... ... because calm and fear cannot exist together ... ... Your thought of calm takes the lead ... ... As soon as you allow it to be there, it spreads out and fear disappears ... ... Fear must disappear because there is only room for calm ... ... Whenever a thought of uncertainty arises, you say ... ... I know my heart is healthy, and that's why I remain calm ... ... and immediately you feel the relaxation of your body, which instantly becomes calmer with this thought ... ... and then you know that your heart is healthy ... ... You help yourself in your waking life ... ... You start your day with conscious and focused thoughts of health ... ... with your special thought ... ... I know my heart is healthy, and that's why I remain calm ... ... every day ... ... every single day ...

You want to feel again that your heart is healthy ... ... because deep inside you know that your heart is truly healthy ... ... So you think ... ... I know my heart is healthy, and that's why I remain calm ... ... This one thought helps you stay calm and trust in the healthy function of your heart ... ... You feel good ... ... Your heart beats steadily and evenly ... ... Your heart is healthy ... ... Every day you can experience this feeling anew ... ... the feeling of calm ... ... the feeling of health ... ... the feeling of a healthy heart ... ... You start your day with conscious and focused thoughts of health ... ... Every day, you experience your healthy heart ...

Hypnosis 2

Today, you have a special goal ... ... You want to trust your heart again ... ... you want to feel deep inside that your heart is healthy ... ... absolutely healthy ... ... You want to let go of fear today and regain self-confidence and trust ... ... You focus on this goal ... ... You want to achieve it today ... ... let go of fear and find self-confidence ... ... feel your healthy heart ... ... You can achieve this today because you can really focus on your goal in trance ... ... so concentrated and targeted ... ... Your goal is clear ... ... Your will is strong ... ... stronger than ever before ... ... You want it more than ever today ... ... you want to let go of the fear for your heart and once again feel your healthy heart naturally and trust it again ... ... Today, you are taking care of it ... ... Today, you are taking care of trusting yourself ... ... and of self-confidence and self-assurance ... ... Today is the most important day in a long time ... ... the day of your liberation ... ... the day of your healthy heart ... ... You free yourself from fear today ... ... Today, you achieve your goal ... ...

trust in yourself ... ... trust in your healthy heart ... ... trust in your healthy heart ...

Now you activate your self-confidence and self-assurance, because these help you let go of the fear for your heart and build new confidence ... ... You succeed because you really embrace it ... ... You have memories of successes within you ... ... You let these memories awaken ... ... and then you can use them to let go of the fear ... ... and trust your heart again ... ... You succeed ... ... In your inner center lies the strength of the successes you've had in your life ... ... You feel it, and now you activate this success power ... ... Now ... ... You activate it with your thoughts ... ... Now ... ... very good ... ... You really succeed ... ... You are activating your own success power at this moment ... ... You are already letting go of fear ... ... You are finding self-confidence and also new courage ... ... Now ... ... Your success power is now actually greater and stronger than ever before ... ... because you are in trance and are activating this power more and more ... ... You achieve your goal ...

Deep within you, you now feel deep calm and your heart beats steadily and evenly ... ... You feel the calmness of your heart ... ... It unfolds more and more, so you become increasingly calm ... ... and trust your heart again ... ... You trust your heart ... ... When you think about your heart now, you remain completely calm and composed ... ... Your heart continues to beat calmly, and you feel completely relaxed ... ... You can now easily imagine that your heart will beat calmly all day and is completely healthy ... ... Just relax even deeper ... ... Let go of all thoughts and breathe slowly and deeply out, then it becomes calmer and calmer within you ... ... And your heart also beats calmly and feels good ... ... It becomes calmer within you ... ... You go even deeper into trance and feel absolutely safe and comfortable ... ... and the calmness connects with your heart, which remains calm and healthy for you now and throughout the day ... ... Your heart is healthy ... ... Your heart beats normally ... ... Your heart is completely healthy and strong ... ... You know that you are healthy and will remain healthy ... ... Fear completely fades away ... ... Fear now completely fades away ... ... It has become meaningless ... ... Calm and trust completely replace fear ... ... Calm and trust and a healthy heart ...

Step by step, the earlier fear is now even being replaced by self-confidence and self-assurance ... ... because you feel the fear leaving and space is becoming available ... ... Finally, you can be free again, leave the house, and feel safe ... ... Self-assurance and self-confidence are now getting stronger ... ... Fear completely disappears, and in its place, self-assurance and self-confidence emerge ... ... anticipation of the next good day ... ... Self-assurance and self-confidence are stronger than you ever thought ... ... You can really feel them now when you dive deep into your feelings ... ... With that, fear completely fades away, and only self-assurance and self-confidence remain ... ... Self-assurance and self-confidence ... ... You did it ... ... You defeated the fear and focused on your successes ... ... That is really excellent because now you can enjoy the day again ... ... free and calm ... ... with self-assurance and self-confidence ... ... You succeed ... ... You really succeed ...

You now feel relaxed and good, and you can truly be proud of having found self-assurance and self-confidence again ... ... You have let go of fear, and you trust your heart again ... ... You really feel good because you did it ... ... You trust your heart again because you are sure it is healthy ...

... This is a special moment ... ... a moment of liberation and strength ... ... You can be very proud of yourself and thank yourself for it ... ... You can also praise yourself because, after all, you have achieved all of this ... ... These are my words you hear ... ... But it is you who turns them into truth ... ... the truth of a healthy heart ... ... Your heart is healthy and beats calmly ...

Very good, a lot has been accomplished today ... ... You know that your heart is healthy and you trust your heart again ... ... This is your success ... ... You can go out again and enjoy the day ... ... It will be easier than you can imagine ... ... and you might even be surprised at how calm you really remain ... ... You will become more composed every day and will handle yourself and your heart with calmness and confidence ... ... In this way, you are successful every day, and your self-confidence and self-assurance become stronger and stronger ... ... You succeed ... ... You have already succeeded ... ... You have truly already succeeded ...

Hypnosis 3

You have a goal, a very specific goal ... ... You want to let go of the fear for your heart, and you want to feel completely healthy again ... ... You want to trust and have confidence in your heart ... ... because your heart is healthy ... ... You've often worried about your heart ... ... But you want to end that because you know your heart is healthy ... ... Sometimes thoughts and worries settle in, making it difficult to find peace ... ... But it can also be easy to return to calm ... ... to natural composure and peace ... ... to the belief in your healthy heart ... ... Today, we're working on doing just that ... ... tuning into yourself and feeling your normal heartbeat ... ... while staying relaxed ... ... consciously and calmly perceiving the natural rhythm of your heart ... ... So, you're setting yourself up for this goal ... ... with your thoughts and with your strength ... ... good ... ... This will succeed ...

You've often tried to fight against the fear and restlessness ... ... Today, it will be different because you want to separate the fear from your heart ... ... so fear and worries can be there, but you relax ... ... All thoughts are allowed, but you keep breathing calmly and evenly ... ... Today, it's about perceiving something different ... ... your hands ... ... and the more you succeed in focusing on the sensation of your hands, the faster the fear separates from your heart ... ... The more you manage to feel your hands today, the faster the fear will separate from your heart ... ... the faster you'll feel the natural health of your heart again ... ... Feel your hands now for a moment ... ... [Wait for ten seconds] ... ... good ...

And now focus on your goal ... ... Until recently, you had fear for your heart ... ... But from now on, it will be like this ... ...

Calm and steady heartbeat with inner composure

... [When stating the goal, feel free to place your palm on the client's solar plexus and then withdraw it. It's not necessary, but it helps a lot, as it "anchors" the goal statement. Of course, you can also incorporate energetic techniques into the hypnosis. Be careful not to repeat the goal.] ...

Now let go of all thoughts and focus your mindfulness on your hands ... ... Let your hands rest relaxed by your sides and feel how they feel ... ... Perhaps they feel quite similar ... ... or one hand is a bit cooler than the other ... ... or warmer ... ... and perhaps it's not so easy to really feel both at the same time, but you can certainly do it ... ...

... ... Maybe it's easier to feel the right hand first and then the left ... ... but over time, you manage to feel both hands at once and concentrate entirely on this perception ... ... because over time, both hands will begin to feel the same ... ... Pay attention to the feeling in your hands and imagine that they feel the same ... ... as if both hands were connected ...

... ... Your thoughts are now only occupied with your relaxed hands ... ... They lie beside your body, and you can sense them ... ... everything else is now unimportant ... ... and it feels good to focus on just one sensation for once ... ... It's all about perception ... ... You don't have to achieve anything right now ... ...

... ... Just be here and feel your hands, that's enough ... ... It's only important to really feel them ... ... and that's what you're doing right now ... ... in this very moment ... ... It's easy and natural for you to consciously perceive your hands and feel their calmness ... ... and if you do feel a slight tension in your hands, just let it go ... ... because right now, it's only about the relaxation of your hands ... ... and you can feel that now ... ... Check if your hands already feel the same ... ... and if not yet, they will in a few moments ...

... ... Now slowly shift your attention from your hands to your arms ... ... through your forearms and upper arms to your shoulders ... ... and from there to your breastbone ... ... and to your heart ... ... good ... ... You can feel it ... ... Everything is calm and relaxed ... ... Your heart is calm and healthy ...

Good ... ... That's enough ... ... Now let your thoughts drift ... ... You don't have to do anything anymore ... ... Your deep inner self has already learned everything ... ... The connection between your heart and fear has been separated ... ... Now, your heart is connected with calm and composure ... ... and your body reflects this through a steady heartbeat ... ... through calm breathing ... ...

… … So, you can come back to calm and relax every day, whenever you want … … simply by focusing on your hands … … both at the same time … … because then the same thing happens as today … … You relax very, very deeply … … and you feel healthy … … Your heart is healthy …

Hypnosis 4

You want to let go of the fear for your heart ... ... You want to enjoy the day again and be completely free ... ... free from any fear ... ... So, you want to trust yourself again ... ... and trust that your heart is healthy ... ... Your mind knows that your heart is healthy ... ... Now, your feelings should learn it again too, so that you can handle yourself with complete ease ... ... You are determined ... ... and because you are so determined to be free again and trust your healthy heart, you will succeed today ... ... Yes, you will succeed today ... ... You end the fear ... ... and you begin to trust ... ... Today ... ... Now ...

Imagine you are in an old theater ... ... A theater like the ones from long ago ... ... with red seats covered in velvet ... ... very soft, sturdy seats ... ... Make yourself comfortable on a velvet-soft red seat. You are the only person in this theater ... ... The entire theater is empty, and it is very quiet here ... ... Let the atmosphere of the theater affect you ... ... The floor is soft as velvet ... ... A very soft carpet ... ... a dark red, just like the covering of the seats ... ... a beautiful, deep red ... ... And from the ceiling hangs a huge chandelier, with a thousand small lights and sparkling crystals ... ... It shines brightly and sparkles and gleams ... ... Make yourself very comfortable in your seat and let yourself feel good ... ... On the walls of the theater hang small lanterns ... ... two or three on each side, right and left ... ... Inside, small, sparkling lights glow ... ... The curtain on the stage is still closed ... ... a thick, dark curtain hides the stage of this old theater ... ... And step by step, it slowly gets darker in the room ... ... The lights are dimmed, and the sparkle softens ... ... It gets darker and darker ... ... And with it, you can let everything inside you become quieter ... ... quieter within you ...

The curtain slowly opens ... ... The heavy, dark curtain silently moves to the side ... ... The curtain opens wider and wider ... ... And it gets darker and darker, quieter and quieter ... ... The curtain opens more and more ... ... But the stage is dark, almost black ... ... The curtain moves silently aside, revealing the entire stage ... ... But everything is dark and black on the stage ... ... You wait in anticipation ... ... What will be on the stage? ... ... What will you see when the light comes on? ... ... When the stage lights up? ... ... And suddenly, the lights come on ... ... Something is written up there ... ... A huge message appears on the stage ... ... In big, bold letters, you see written ...

I release all fear and move into trust.

I trust in my healthy heart.

... [Read the affirmation slowly and a little louder than the previous text to highlight it a bit. Then, pause for about 30 seconds before continuing.] ...

Let these wise words flow into your innermost being ... ... let them work and take effect ... ... Allow yourself a time of calm and mindfulness ... ... calm and mindfulness ... ... and feel your steady heartbeat ... ... because now you are truly calm inside, and your heart beats just as calmly and evenly ... ... Now, any possibility of fear dissolves, and you become calm ... ... Everything you can feel and experience in a state of hypnosis, you can also feel and experience when you are fully awake ... ... That is possible ... ... That is truly possible ... ... if it aligns with your own inner goals ... ... and you have this goal, to let go of fear forever ... ... You have this goal, to trust your heart again ... ... to trust again that your heart beats calmly and evenly ... ... just like now ... ... all day long, just like now ... ... Fear should dissolve ... ... Fear should fade away ... ... Trust should arise ... ... Trust should remain ... ... Maybe you can already feel the new trust within you now ... ... or perhaps you will feel it in a few minutes as your affirmation unfolds even more ... ... because it will ... ... It unfolds and becomes stronger until it turns into your truly new and stable belief ... ... your new attitude of trust in your healthy heart ... ... because that is what you have ... ... a healthy heart ... ... a truly healthy heart ...

The words you could read on the stage of the theater are deeply ingrained ... ... they flow into your innermost being and become your truth ... ... Look at the stage again and read once more what is written there because it is deeply written within you ...

I release all fear and move into trust.

I trust in my healthy heart.

... ... Now allow yourself to simply rest ... ... without needing to think or do anything ... ... Just be there and breathe in and out ... ... calmly in and out ... ... because with the flow of your breath, the effect of the words flows deeper into your inner being ...

Good ... ... You have achieved a lot ... ... Whenever you want, you can repeat the affirmation every morning after waking up, if you wish ... ... and each time, the new belief in your healthy heart will become more stable and natural ... ... Your heart is healthy ... ... Your heart is healthy ... ... quite naturally ...

Hypnosis 5

You have a clear goal ... ... a very important goal ... ... You want to trust your heart again and live your day without fear ... ... You know the fear of heart disease or sudden cardiac arrest ... ... But this fear should end now ... ... because now you can tune in to freedom and calmness within yourself again ... ... You can be free again and enjoy the day ... ... trust your heart completely once more ... ... Today, you can use the path of trance ... ... You are already in trance ... ... and therefore it is also possible to find help deep within you ... ... in your subconscious ... ... more help than you think ... ... Now you are calm and relaxed, free from fear ... ... and now you can communicate with your subconscious and decide what should be ... ... Your subconscious supports you because it hears and understands my words, which today become your own ... ... So, you say to yourself inside ...

... ... I can and will trust my heart again ... ... because I know it is healthy and beats evenly ...

… … I can and will trust my heart again … … because I know that trust helps me more than anything else …

… … I can and will trust my heart again … … because I know that self-confidence also means confidence in my heart …

… … I can and will trust my heart again … … because I know that with it, I will succeed and overcome fear …

… … That's what matters … … That's really what matters …

… … I always remember that my heart has actually always been healthy and has always beaten normally … … so I also know that it will continue to beat normally …

… … I always remember that my heart has actually always been healthy and has always beaten normally … … so I can trust that it will continue to do so …

… … I always remember that my heart has actually always been healthy and has always beaten normally … … so I can also remain calm and always return to calm …

…… I always remember that my heart has actually always been healthy and has always beaten normally …… so I also know that I am healthy …

…… That's what matters …… That's really what matters …

…… I feel that my heart is beating calmly at this moment …… and that helps me always feel that my heart is okay …

…… I feel that my heart is beating calmly at this moment …… and that shows me clearly that my heart will always be reliable …

…… I feel that my heart is beating calmly at this moment …… and my heartbeat always returns to this calmness …

…… I feel that my heart is beating calmly at this moment …… and this physical calm helps me remain inwardly calm …

…… That's what matters …… That's really what matters …

…… I feel free, and I am inwardly completely relaxed and calm …… and I maintain this inner calmness and feel it every day …

… … I feel free, and I am inwardly completely relaxed and calm … … and I know that any excitement will quickly pass …

… … I feel free, and I am inwardly completely relaxed and calm … … and any acceleration of my heartbeat is natural and will calm down again …

… … I feel free, and I am inwardly completely relaxed and calm … … and I remain calm and composed even when my heart beats faster …

… … That's what matters … … That's really what matters …

… … I give myself the freedom to leave the house every day and be among people … … because I know that my heart will beat calmly for me …

… … I give myself the freedom to leave the house every day and be among people … … because that's how I regain self-confidence …

… … I give myself the freedom to leave the house every day and be among people … … because I am stronger than any thought of fear …

... ... I give myself the freedom to leave the house every day and be among people ... ... because that's how I take control of my life again ...

... ... That's what matters ... ... That's really what matters ...

Good ... ... You have already achieved a lot ... ... Now let the words you've heard flow deep into your innermost being ... ... because there they become truth ... ... they are already truth there ... ... Everything you have heard becomes what you say to yourself with your inner voice, with your inner will ... ... You know deep within that your heart is healthy ... ... and that's exactly what you can feel again ... ... You feel that your heart is healthy and always beats in the way that is best for you ...

Hypnosis 6

Instructions for Implementation

In this hypnosis session, an anchor will be used. An anchor (or trigger) is a stimulus that creates a specific feeling or evokes a particular thought. It's a signal that the client perceives and then triggers an inner process. The established anchor then replaces the suggestion. In everyday life, a client can use an anchor to trigger or establish a desired state, even without being in a trance state. Many stimuli can be used as anchors/triggers. I work with the following possibilities, which I also use in the series "Ten Hypnoses":

- Physical anchors (clenching the hand, pressing the ball of the thumb ...)
- Visual anchors (symbols, word cards ...)
- Acoustic anchors (signal noises like a phone ring, melodies ...)
- Olfactory anchors (scent oils ...)
- Haptic anchors (comfort objects, talismans ...)

I also distinguish between perihypnotic and post-hypnotic anchors. Perihypnotic anchors are mainly used during hypnosis when the therapist sets up the anchor and then triggers it repeatedly as a supplement to suggestions and visualizations. Post-hypnotic anchors are primarily set up for use after the session so that the client can help themselves with them. Have a card ready with the inscription, "My heart is healthy and beats evenly because everything is fine." and discuss before hypnosis that you will hand the card to the client during the session. They don't need to open their eyes. Simply announce a touch once again shortly before handing over the card and touch the client's hand with it so that they can grasp it. Just follow the instructions in the text!

+++ End of instructions +++

Today, I'm setting up an anchor for you … … It's a very effective tool that makes it easy for you to quickly feel the calm rhythm of your heartbeat … … Whenever you feel like your heart is starting to race, you will feel with the help of your anchor that your heart is actually beating calmly and evenly … … You know it has always just felt like your heart was racing ... ... In reality, it beats slowly at times and a bit faster at other times, but always evenly and normally ... ... The key is to quickly feel that your heart is beating normally when you're nervous ... ... It's a simple thought that can help you ... ... It's the thought ... ... My heart is healthy and beats evenly because everything is fine ... ... You want to anchor this thought so that the old fear doesn't even have a chance to arise ... ... With this firmly anchored thought, you are calm within yourself, and your heart beats so gently that you don't even think about it anymore ... ... Deep inside, you trust again that your heart is healthy and that you are healthy ... ... and will remain healthy ... ... So, let's set up your anchor so that you can use it anytime ...

But first, it's all about a beautiful calm ... ... because deep in calm and relaxation, it's much easier to anchor new thoughts ... ... and let go of fear ... ... A feeling of freedom and trust arises ... ... Now you feel the relaxation ... ... You are in a pleasant and comfortable trance and feel free and healthy ... ... You feel your heart beating calmly ... ... It feels completely calm ... ... calm and healthy ... ... perhaps so calm that you can't even feel the individual heartbeats ... ... or just barely, because everything is really okay ... ... You focus on the feeling of calm ... ... The more you can feel the calm of the moment now, the better and faster your anchor can be set ... ... Now, you don't have to worry about anything ... ... Now you don't have to do anything and don't have to achieve anything ... ... Now, you have calm ... ... Now you also feel calm ... ... Now, you can enjoy calm ... ... just enjoy calm ...

Now, in this pleasant relaxation, it's easy to feel that your heart is healthy and beating healthily ... ... This is already much better than before ... ... You accept yourself at this moment and feel healthy ... ... The more clearly you can feel the relaxation now, the better you can also feel that you are healthy ... ... that your heart is healthy ... ... So feel the relaxation and feel your healthy heart ... ... Now ... ... Now it works ... ... You can feel calm and health ... ... Now, I'm giving you the card in your hand ... ... [Touch the client's hand and hand them the card. They can keep their eyes closed.] ... ... Feel the card in your hand ... ... You know what's written on it ... ... it says ... ... My heart is healthy and beats evenly because everything is fine ... ... You think about this sentence, this attitude ... ... You feel that everything is truly fine ... ... You recognize that you are truly healthy ... ... that your heart is truly healthy ... ... The card becomes a switch for you ... ... As soon as you look at it, read the sentence on it, it becomes your truth, deeply ingrained ... ... The card reminds you that you are healthy and that your heart is healthy ... ... It helps you because whenever you carry it with you, it gives you calm and confidence ... ... it's enough that you carry it with you because your subconscious has stored the card as a signal of your safety ... ... as a signal of health ... ... And whenever even the feeling of fear could arise, you take the card back in your hand and read what's on it ... ... My heart is healthy and beats evenly because everything is fine ... ... and immediately you feel calm and confidence deep within you again ... ... and you feel your heartbeat calming down ... ... as calm as now ... ... just as calm as now ... ... with just one look at the card ... ... even when you hold the card in your hand or touch it without reading it, you immediately find calm and confidence ... ... just like today ... ... every day, just like today ...

Hypnosis 7

You know the fear for your heart, and you know it isn't logically justified ... ... But fear is a feeling and doesn't need logic ... ... At the same time, you know that your heart is healthy and that the fear for your heart doesn't concern any real danger ... ... That's why you can also work on changing your feelings ... ... It may not seem simple ... ... and yet it's possible and often easier than you think to change your own feelings ... ... On closer inspection, it's not really the feeling of fear but an inexplicable, not yet fully grasped feeling ... ... and such feelings are then judged as fear ... ... Fear is sometimes a judgment, a thought ... ... That's how it is with the fear for your heart and the fear of cardiac arrest or sudden death ... ... You know this fear ... ... A racing heartbeat that suddenly becomes so noticeable that you think your heart is racing out of control ... ... In reality, it beats slower than it feels at that moment ... ... So today, it's about strengthening your body awareness ... ... making sure you perceive your heartbeat just as it really is ... ... and at the same time, instructing your body to calm your heart ...

… now and always … … Now, your heart is calm and beats evenly … … This state helps your body learn to calm down quickly … … to quickly enter this state … … and to stay in it …

Now breathe in deeply and exhale slowly and for a long time so that you become even calmer … … [In the client's breathing rhythm, please!] … … deep in … … and out … … and in … … and out … … in … … out … … in … … out … … Good … … With each breath, you become calmer … … Your heart beats calmly and evenly … … And now feel the calmness of your body very consciously … … Feel the pleasant calm … … Feel your feet first … … Your feet carry you all day, but now they too can rest … … Your feet are completely calm … … and this calmness slowly flows into your legs … … Your legs are calm and relaxed … … Your legs are completely relaxed … … The calves are relaxed, and you feel this calmness and relaxation … … Your body should always feel this relaxed … … Your entire body should always be this calm … … And this calmness flows further into your thighs … … With each breath, this gentle calmness flows further from your feet into your legs … … Your legs are completely calm and relaxed … … and become calmer with each breath ... ... calmer and calmer ... ... and the pleasant and relaxed feeling flows up into your upper body ... ... Your belly relaxes further, and your back also feels the relaxation rising from your feet to the top ... ... Now focus on your hands ... ... Your hands are also completely relaxed ... ... lying loosely by your side ... ... and each finger feels the relaxation ... ... Each finger is deeply relaxed and calm ... ... And this beautiful calmness flows from your fingers through your hands into your arms ... ... Your forearms are relaxed ... ... You feel the relaxation of the forearms with each breath more clearly ... ... Completely relaxed fingers and completely relaxed hands ... ... and completely relaxed forearms ... ... And from there, the relaxation flows into your upper arms and shoulders ... ... You feel the relaxation from your fingertips to your shoulders ... ... From the outside, the calm and relaxation of the body slowly flow inward ... ... from outside to inside ... ... Calmness flows slowly from your toes through your calves to your thighs ... ... from there into your belly and back ... ... And from your fingertips, calmness flows through your hands ... ... to your forearms and into your upper arms ... ... Further to your shoulders ... ... and from there to your heart ... ... So all the calm and relaxation that you can feel in your body flows from outside to inside ... ... from your feet to your heart ... ... from your fingertips to your heart ... ... and finally, you feel calm and relaxation throughout your entire body ...

... ... Your heart beats calmly and evenly ... ... completely calmly and evenly ... ... because calmness flows from outside to inside ... ... Your body stores this path for you now ... ... Your body is training right now to always let calmness and relaxation flow from outside to inside to your heart ... ... Whenever fear could arise ... ... Immediately, your body sends every bit of relaxation it can find from outside to inside to your heart ... ... So, your heartbeat immediately becomes calmer ... ... just like now ... ... So, you yourself immediately become calmer in your thoughts and feelings ... ... just like now ... ... calmer and more composed ... ... just like now ... ... And then you feel that your heart beats calmly and steadily ... ... calmly and steadily ... ... just like now ... ... Your heart beats evenly and healthily ... ... just like now ... ... You can trust your body because it acts for you in the same way every time ... ... Your body repeatedly sends calmness and relaxation from outside to inside to your heart ... ... because there are always body parts that are relaxed, always ... ... and from all these relaxed areas, your body sends calmness and relaxation to your heart ... ... So, your heart always beats evenly and at just the right pace that's good for you ... ... Your body ensures this natural balance because you allow it now ... ... and your body always ensures this balance and lets calmness and relaxation flow from outside to inside ... ... always and every day ... ... always and every day ...

You can let go of all thoughts, you don't have to hold onto anything in your mind because your body has already understood how to do it ... ... Your body knows how to restore balance ... ... Your body is already set to send signals of calmness and relaxation from outside to inside to your heart whenever you get agitated or a fearful thought arises ... ... and your heart remains calm ... ... Your heart remains truly calm ... ... And you remain inwardly calm and composed ... ... You trust your healthy heart ... ... because it also feels healthy to you again ... ... Healthy calmness in a healthy heart ... ... healthy calmness in your healthy heart ... ... Now ...

Hypnosis 8

Instructions for Implementation

In this hypnosis session, ideomotor responses are used. Ideomotor response refers to the phenomenon where our body movements reflect our feelings and thoughts. In everyday life, this following is shown through body posture, muscle tension, and movement patterns of a person, which naturally change with mood and thoughts. In trance, ideomotor signals can be used to obtain information that the client cannot actively share. For example, the subconscious can answer questions with an agreed finger signal. Of course, ideomotor responses can also be used suggestively, such as with arm levitations and catalepsies. An ideomotor approach strengthens trust in hypnosis and in one's own ability to change and thus supports the therapy.

+++ End of instructions +++

You want to let go of the fear ... ... You know your heart is healthy, but somehow fear has settled there ... ... But today, you can separate the fear from your heart again ... ... You can take it away and let it go ... ... This happens in two steps ... ... First, you detach the fear from your heart, and then you let it go completely, so it disappears entirely ... ... For this, I invite your subconscious to work with me and with you ... ... With the help of your subconscious, you will succeed in removing the fear today ... ... Your subconscious can help you and more ... ... It can show you that it has detached and let go of the fear ... ... and you might wonder how that can happen ... ... You will experience it in just a few moments ...

Imagine for a moment that your subconscious could make your arm feel light ... ... so light that your arm rises into the air as if weightless ... ... If your subconscious can do that, it can also separate the fear from your heart for you ... ... So, I'm now agreeing with your subconscious as follows: The separation of the fear from your heart will be shown by your subconscious placing your right hand on your heart ... ... as a sign of inner change ... ... The agreement is set because your subconscious has understood me ... ... Now imagine that your subconscious moves your right arm ... ... Your right arm becomes very light and is lifted by your subconscious ... ... Step by step ... ... Just let it happen, then your right arm will move as if by itself ... ... Your arm is slowly lifted ... ... rising up, feather-light ... ... and you don't have to do anything for it, you don't have to help your arm ... ... Your arm moves upward ...

[Please be patient. The suggestive request leads to the arm slowly rising. This may take a few minutes, but it will happen. First, the arm should move slightly upward. Then please suggest the movement toward the heart.]

... ... And now your subconscious grabs hold of the fear to detach it ... ... Your hand moves toward your heart ... ... Your hand moves toward your heart and will rest on your heart in just a few moments ... ... Your hand moves toward your heart ... ... and as soon as your hand touches your body, the fear is detached ... ... separated from your heart ... ... Your hand rests firmly and steadily on your heart ... ... Your hand rests firmly and steadily on your heart ...

[Stay with it until the hand lies flat and with some pressure on the client's body, in the heart area. This is as simple an ideomotor response as an arm levitation.]

... ... Good ... ... very good ... ... Your hand has placed itself on your body without your help ... ... Your body did that for you ... ... Your subconscious controlled that ... ... The first step is done ...

... ... Now, feel your hand on your body ... ... This is the sign, the signal from your subconscious ... ... Now the fear is being separated from your heart ... ... Now the fear is really being detached from your heart ... ... This happens deep within you, and your subconscious shows you each step with the movement of your hand ... ... The first step is complete because your hand rests on your heart ... ... Now the fear is being released ... ... It flows from the heart into the hand ... ... Maybe you feel a slight tingling or some warmth in your hand because now the fear is being released and flows into the hand ... ... or it feels completely normal because you are so relaxed now that you are only concerned with pleasant thoughts and sensations ... ... Now the fear is separated from you ... ... Your hand grabs the fear ... ... You feel the hand on your body ... ... The fear is separated from the heart ... ... The hand grabs the fear ... ... Now, the next step can follow ... ... Letting go of the fear ... ... Your body will also show you this step ... ... because again, your hand will move ...

You have already achieved a lot ... ... Your fear has indeed already been separated from your heart ... ... Now your body can completely let go of the fear ... ... For this, your arm now moves away from your body again ... ... The hand releases the contact with your body, and the arm is lifted again ... ... Your subconscious does this for you ... ... Your arm is lifted and moves back to your side ... ... Your arm becomes mobile and sinks onto the surface, next to your body ... ... Your arm does this at exactly the speed your subconscious needs to completely let go of the fear ...

[Stay with it, if necessary, add some suggestions. The arm will follow the suggestive request and move to the side of the body and become relaxed and mobile again.]

... ... Good ... ... That's right ... ... Your arm reaches the surface, and the fear disappears forever ... ... The fear disappears forever ...

Now everything is good ... ... The fear is released, and you have let it go ... ... From now on, you feel the health of your heart ... ... From now on, you remain calm and composed and know that your heart is healthy ... ... because the fear is over ... ... has disappeared ... ... Self-confidence and self-assurance unfold within you and spread ... ... Self-assurance and trust are now connected with your heart ... ... Trust in the heart ... ... Trust in your heart ... ... deep trust, deep in your heart ... ... Now ...

Hypnosis 9

Instructions for Implementation

A self-hypnosis trigger is a signal that initiates the state of trance. With its help, even an inexperienced client can continue working with self-hypnosis at home. Of course, they can "only" work with simple suggestions that they can easily remember and that we should prepare, or with simple visualizations. Triggered self-hypnosis is a very good tool to give the client a task and support the therapy. So, the time between sessions in the practice is not without therapy but is continued at home. Completely self-directed self-hypnosis, without a trigger, is also easily learnable but takes a lot of time and practice. Setting up the trigger is a fairly simple task and of course, relieves the client, who I do not want to burden with the training of a self-directed self-hypnosis. Despite some skeptics, I also claim here that there is really no problem in teaching a client simple trigger self-hypnosis. It is no more dangerous than meditation, autogenic training, or yoga. You can survive that unscathed at home as well. I have experienced numerous patients in my practice who not only handled self-hypnosis well but enjoyed it. And if a patient enjoys doing self-hypnosis, no matter how simple the suggestion may seem, that's a very good support for compliance. Discuss the process once before hypnosis and give the client a short list of steps for self-hypnosis as a small guide.

+++ End of instructions +++

Now we will prepare self-hypnosis together because you can use self-hypnosis to tune into calmness and security every day ... ... to find trust in your heart and be sure that your heart is healthy ... ... Self-hypnosis is simple if we prepare it here together, and that's what we're doing ... ... Each self-hypnosis helps you let go of fear and feel secure again ... ... Now focus on the feeling of relaxation ... ... a good and comfortable and secure feeling ... ... calm and composed yet very normal, very natural ... ... You can come into this state yourself and then use it ... ... It is indeed simple ... ... We are doing it together now ... ... Feel how comfortable it is to be inwardly so calm ...

You can create this trance yourself ... ... anywhere, even at home ... ... For this, you simply do the following ... ... You close your eyes and breathe consciously and calmly in and out ... ... and you whisper as you inhale ... ... I breathe in ... ... As you exhale, you whisper ... ... I breathe out and go into trance ... ... and you repeat this until you get tired ... ... Always make sure to whisper when inhaling and exhaling ... ... It works well; you can try it out in a few minutes ... ... Repeat this until you truly become tired ... ... it happens very quickly ... ... Make yourself as comfortable as possible ... ... Then close your eyes and begin your ritual ... ... Pay conscious attention to the rhythm of your breathing and whisper ... ... I breathe in ... ... I breathe out and go into trance ... ... I breathe in ... ... I breathe out and go into trance ... ... and very quickly, you will become tired and actually go into a pleasant trance ...

After that, you can deepen the trance so that you can relax even deeper ... ... This is also very simple ... ... Whisper ten times ... ... I am now going deeper into trance ... ... and count to ten as you do ... ... It goes like this ... ... I am now going deeper into trance once ... ... I am now going deeper into trance twice ... ... I am now going deeper into trance three times ... ... and so on ... ... until you finally reach ten and whisper ... ... I am now going deeper into trance ten times ... ... and with each repetition and with each count, you actually go deeper into trance ... ... On the one hand, you stay awake enough to keep speaking and guiding your self-hypnosis ... ... On the other hand, you also go into a deep trance ... ... That really works simultaneously ...

[For deepening and the main part, I recommend counting with the suggestions ... once ... twice, etc. This has the advantage that the client is not distracted by the question of how many times they have now repeated the suggestion. It doesn't really matter if it's ten repetitions; in trance, they can more easily keep the thread this way. Of course, you can also speak all ten repetitions for the client. After all, you are also working suggestively in this hypnosis. It's not just self-hypnosis training but a hypnosis session.]

Then follows the important part of the suggestion ... ... You use a self-suggestion that helps your subconscious let go of fear anytime, even before it really comes up ... ... and the suggestion helps you quickly get into a truly calm and confident state again ... ... You also whisper the suggestion ten times ... ... You say ten times ... ... My heart is healthy, and I remain completely calm ... ... Remember to always count ... ... So say ... ... My heart is healthy, and I remain completely calm once ... ... My heart is healthy, and I remain completely calm twice ... ... My heart is healthy, and I remain completely calm three times ... ... and finally ... ... My heart is healthy, and I remain completely calm ten times ... ... and then you may enjoy the calm ...

Then comes the exit, which you can also do yourself ... ... It's simple because your subconscious has learned it for you ... Imagine there's a draft, and it gets really cold ... ... Then say loudly and clearly ... ... I'm coming back now and waking up ... ... then count quickly and loudly to three and open your eyes ... ... You can do it, so once again ... ... To wake up, imagine a draft ... ... and then say with a strong voice ... ... I'm coming back now and waking up – One – Two – Three ... ... and then you're suddenly wide awake and can open your eyes ... ... It's that simple ...

You have learned and understood how to do self-hypnosis ... ... You can now do a self-hypnosis and work on trusting your heart again ... ... Your subconscious has learned for you to help you ... ... Your breathing brings you into trance, which you deepen with the words ... I am now going deeper into trance ... Then follows your suggestion ... My heart is healthy, and I remain completely calm ... and at the end, imagine a draft and say ... I'm coming back now and waking up – One – Two – Three ...

Hypnosis 10

There is a very special place that you can imagine ... ... it's the land of dreams ... ... This land of dreams awaits you ... ... It is in a secret place that only you can go to ... ... secret but very close ... ... Focus on the center of your body, on the solar plexus, and direct all your attention there ... ... Dive with all your attention through the solar plexus into your body ... ... sink deeper and deeper into yourself with each breath ... ... deeper with each breath ... ... With that, you can feel and see deeper than you think ... ... You dive into the deepest world of your own creativity and imagination ... ... into the land of your dreams ... ... Perhaps you know that dream and reality are only a breath apart ...

You are standing in the middle of an old road ... ... a road with some rough spots and potholes ... ... It's the road of fear that you've been walking on for so long ... ... But in the land of dreams, there is no fear ... ... here, there are only images of it ... ... memories that you can view and understand ... ... Nothing can harm you here ... ... Here, your heart beats completely calmly and evenly ... ... So, you can walk on this road today ... ... Your goal in the land of dreams is always yourself ... ... nothing else can be found here but yourself ... ... and that's why the road of fear is also safe here ... ... So, you start walking on the road of fear, which leads you through the land of dreams, past images that show you something about yourself and your fear of your heart ... ... They show you how it was so often in the fearful moments, in the moments when the fear of sudden death suddenly struck and took hold of you ... ... You've experienced that often, very often ... ... years ago already, but also in more recent times ... ... On this journey, you are accompanied by a person of your choice, who can or could comfort you especially well if a sudden panic attack occurs in your everyday life and that person were with you ... ... Whoever comes to mind or appears before your inner eye ... ... Let yourself be accompanied by this person ... ... Let them help you today in the land of dreams because that is why they are here ... ... to help you ... ... to help you now ...

... ... The first thing you come to is an image that shows you how you once had a panic attack while out and about, on an open road or in a crowd ... ... All of a sudden, your heart started racing, and the fear was there, you couldn't do anything about it ... ... maybe people stared at you, maybe you didn't even notice because you were busy with yourself and your survival ... ... at least it felt like you were suffocating or dying ... ... You thought your heart was going to stop, and you would die ... ... You see it again as if in a still image ... ... and the comforter who is now with you takes you in their arms and tells you it wasn't your fault, you didn't do, think, or say anything wrong ... ... It was never your fault ... ... and then you take yourself in your arms too, comforting yourself for the suffering in fear and for the suffering of earlier times, even if earlier suffering had nothing to do with fear ... ... Then, this image of the unpleasant situation dissolves before your eyes because it has long since outlived its usefulness ... ... You don't need it anymore ... ... Then you continue walking, accompanied by your comforter, and come to an image that shows you what you've felt most guilty about or still feel guilty about today ... ... perhaps an image that has nothing to do with your fear of your heart, at least not at first glance ... ... maybe you see something here that you missed ... ... something you did and later thought you shouldn't have done ... ... or wished could be undone ... ... But that's not possible; it happened as it did, and nothing and no one can ever undo it, just as everything that happened in your life can never be undone …

… … The person who comforts you takes you in their arms here too and holds you close, comforting you for your pain and suffering … … for the guilt and your feelings of guilt so that you can let them go … … Then you take yourself in your arms to comfort yourself for all the burdens and hardships you've had to carry up to now … … You come to a spring where fresh water bubbles up … … You hear the sound of the bubbling water and sit by this spring … … You dip your hands into the pleasantly cool water … … Today, you may wash your hands in innocence … … You cleanse your hands until you feel you can now let go of your feelings of guilt … … The land of dreams tells you today that most of the difficulties in our lives come from feelings that were never truly our own … … So, a large part of our feelings of guilt was not born within us but in the feelings we once believed were ours or still believe to be … … But they are just false feelings … … Many times in your life, you've felt guilty or had a bad conscience … … Deep inside, you feel that it was mostly because you were once told that you were guilty ... ... So, you even felt guilty because you were afraid for your heart ... ... because others couldn't understand it ... ... You let go of these feelings of guilt now ... ... Your comforter helps you to let go of all these old thoughts of guilt and feelings of guilt that were never your own and to feel free again ... ... to feel again that your heart is healthy ...

You breathe deeply in and out, and it becomes clear to you that it was the old feelings of guilt that allowed this fear to come into being ... ... Deep down, you once believed you had to be punished, but the land of dreams knows no punishments ... ... Here, you meet yourself with openness and affection ... ... Affection that your comforter has for you ... ... Affection that you have for yourself ... ... You meet yourself with self-love ... ... with love from you to you ... ... Love from you to you ... ... You continue walking and think about how the land of dreams truly exists ... ... it lies deep within you ... ... It has always been there ... ... I'm just telling you about it ...

All Titles in the Series

Volume 1: Smoking Cessation
Volume 2: Anxiety and Restlessness
Volume 3: Burnout
Volume 4: Reducing Overweight
Volume 5: Coping with the Past
Volume 6: Suicidal Thoughts and Attempts
Volume 7: Psycho-Oncology
Volume 8: Obsessions and Tics
Volume 9: Self-Confidence and Decision-Making
Volume 10: Grief Work
Volume 11: Psychosomatics
Volume 12: Chronic Pain
Volume 13: Depressive Thoughts
Volume 14: Panic Attacks
Volume 15: Domestic Violence, Victim Support
Volume 16: Post-Traumatic Stress
Volume 17: Exam Anxiety and Stage Fright
Volume 18: Anti-Violence Training, Offender Support
Volume 19: Addiction Tendencies
Volume 20: Social Phobia and Fear of Contact
Volume 21: Nail Biting
Volume 22: Self-Awareness and Self-Love
Volume 23: Teeth Grinding and Night Clenching
Volume 24: Feelings of Guilt
Volume 25: Fear in Crowds
Volume 26: Fear of Flying, Aviophobia
Volume 27: Fear in Enclosed Spaces, Claustrophobia
Volume 28: Tinnitus, Ear Noises
Volume 29: Fear of Heights
Volume 30: Neurodermatitis

Volume 31: Finding Inner Balance
Volume 32: Overcoming Loneliness
Volume 33: Fear of Illness, Hypochondria
Volume 34: Anticipatory Anxiety, Fear of Fear
Volume 35: Jealousy in Relationships
Volume 36: Driving Anxiety
Volume 37: New Start after Separation
Volume 38: Fear of Injections
Volume 39: Heart Anxiety Neurosis
Volume 40: Overcoming Resentment and Anger
Volume 41: Resolving Blockages and Positive Thinking
Volume 42: Stress Reduction, Stress Management
Volume 43: Body Relaxation
Volume 44: Deep Relaxation
Volume 45: Fear of the Dark
Volume 46: Falling Asleep and Staying Asleep
Volume 47: Compulsive Buying
Volume 48: Restless Legs Syndrome
Volume 49: Bulimia
Volume 50: Anorexia
Volume 51: Overcoming Nightmares
Volume 52: Imagined Deformity
Volume 53: Overcoming Distrust, Finding Trust
Volume 54: Processing Failures
Volume 55: Humiliation, Emotional Hurt
Volume 56: Distressing Compassion, Vicarious Suffering
Volume 57: Self-Forgiveness
Volume 58: Self-Awareness, Self-Confidence
Volume 59: Saying No
Volume 60: Assertiveness
Volume 61: Setting Boundaries and Self-Assertion
Volume 62: Decision-Making Ability

Volume 63: Success Orientation
Volume 64: Ruminating, Circular Thinking
Volume 65: Accepting Pregnancy
Volume 66: Birth Preparation
Volume 67: Spiritual Opening
Volume 68: Joy of Life and Inner Lightness
Volume 69: Patience and Inner Peace
Volume 70: Fibromyalgia and Rheumatism
Volume 71: Irritable Bowel Syndrome, Crohn's Disease
Volume 72: Fear of Nausea, Emetophobia
Volume 73: Stuttering and Cluttering, Speech Flow Disorders
Volume 74: Concentration and Knowledge Anchoring
Volume 75: Vitality and Spontaneity
Volume 76: Searching for Meaning and Finding Goals
Volume 77: Life Crises, Life Events
Volume 78: Workaholism, Goal Obsession
Volume 79: Helper Syndrome, Helpless Helpers
Volume 80: Medication Abuse
Volume 81: Gambling Addiction
Volume 82: Internet Addiction, Smartphone Addiction
Volume 83: Hoarding Disorder, Compulsive Collecting
Volume 84: Conspiracy Thoughts, Overvalued Ideas
Volume 85: Fear of Operations and Treatments
Volume 86: Fear of Aging
Volume 87: Travel Anxiety
Volume 88: Anxiety When Urinating, Paruresis
Volume 89: Fear of Intimacy and Togetherness
Volume 90: Fear of Blushing
Volume 91: Coming Out in Homosexuality
Volume 92: Charisma Training
Volume 93: Migraines and Chronic Headaches
Volume 94: Overcoming Allergies, Bronchial Asthma

Volume 95: Normalizing Blood Pressure
Volume 96: Compulsive Perfectionism
Volume 97: Sports Hypnosis, Motivation
Volume 98: Sports Hypnosis, Performance Enhancement
Volume 99: Determination and Focus
Volume 100: Encountering the Inner Child
Volume 101: Cravings, Binge Eating
Volume 102: Stimulating Metabolism
Volume 103: Bipolar Mood Swings
Volume 104: Borderline, Identity Crises
Volume 105: Hypomania, Euphoria, Mania
Volume 106: Restlessness, Agitation
Volume 107: Nervous Breakdown
Volume 108: Adjustment Disorders
Volume 109: Self-Alienation, Depersonalization
Volume 110: Ending Self-Pity
Volume 111: Primary Gain of Illness
Volume 112: Secondary Gain of Illness
Volume 113: Bullying, Victim Support
Volume 114: Letting Go of Envy and Jealousy
Volume 115: Fear of Spiders, Arachnophobia
Volume 116: Fear of Dogs or Cats
Volume 117: Fear of Strangers, Xenophobia
Volume 118: Excessive Worries, Generalized Anxiety
Volume 119: Strengthening Sense of Responsibility
Volume 120: Unrequited Love, Heartache
Volume 121: Work-Life Balance
Volume 122: Letting Go of Unattainable Goals
Volume 123: Allowing and Accepting Help
Volume 124: Letting Go of Adult Children
Volume 125: Tourette Syndrome
Volume 126: Life Changes and New Starts

Volume 127: Accepting Life in a Wheelchair
Volume 128: Understanding and Overcoming Homesickness
Volume 129: Understanding and Overcoming Wanderlust
Volume 130: Dizziness, Meniere's Disease
Volume 131: Overcoming Aggression
Volume 132: Cutting and Self-Harm
Volume 133: Hair Pulling, Trichotillomania
Volume 134: Postpartum Depression
Volume 135: For Relatives of Dementia Patients
Volume 136: Self-Harm, Artificial Disorders
Volume 137: Activating Self-Healing Powers
Volume 138: Preventing Depression Relapse
Volume 139: Reactive Psychoses, Follow-Up
Volume 140: Obsessive Thoughts and Impulses
Volume 141: Compulsive Checking
Volume 142: Compulsive Counting, Symmetry Obsession
Volume 143: Compulsive Washing, Cleanliness Obsession
Volume 144: Compulsive Questioning
Volume 145: Dissociative Paralysis
Volume 146: Phantom Pain
Volume 147: Overcoming Complaining
Volume 148: Hay Fever, Pollen Allergy
Volume 149: Sexual Abuse, Victim Support
Volume 150: Standing Strong Against Sexism, #metoo
Volume 151: Binge Eating
Volume 152: Overcoming Thoughts of Revenge
Volume 153: Detachment from the Aggressor, Stockholm Syndrome
Volume 154: Courage to Separate
Volume 155: Chronic Fatigue, Exhaustion
Volume 156: Fear of the Future, Existential Anxiety
Volume 157: Excessive Worry About Children
Volume 158: Fear of Failure

Volume 159: Ending Distrust and Control
Volume 160: Dejection, Dysphoria
Volume 161: Boreout, Chronic Boredom
Volume 162: Bipolar Disorders, Relapse Prevention
Volume 163: Mania, Relapse Prevention
Volume 164: Nihilism, Feelings of Worthlessness
Volume 165: Thumb Sucking
Volume 166: Being Brave
Volume 167: Being Proud
Volume 168: Overcoming Shyness
Volume 169: Being Able to Delegate Responsibility
Volume 170: Being Able to Show Emotions
Volume 171: Letting Go of Guilt, Victim Support
Volume 172: Processing Guilt, Offender Support
Volume 173: Mood Swings, Cyclothymia
Volume 174: Lack of Drive, Vital Sadness
Volume 175: Hearing Voices with Reality Reference
Volume 176: Confident Communication
Volume 177: Standing Up for Oneself
Volume 178: Taking New Paths
Volume 179: Confident Job Application
Volume 180: No Longer Being Taken Advantage Of
Volume 181: End of Submissiveness
Volume 182: Depressive Numbness
Volume 183: Mood Drops, Affective Incontinence
Volume 184: Mood Instability
Volume 185: Somatoform Disorders
Volume 186: Stomach Ulcer, Psychosomatic
Volume 187: Accepting Amputation
Volume 188: Overcoming and Letting Go of Hatred
Volume 189: Ending Accusations
Volume 190: Allowing Tears, Being Able to Cry

Volume 191: Finding and Sorting Repressed Feelings
Volume 192: Somatoform Pain
Volume 193: Living Autonomously
Volume 194: Anhedonia, Joylessness
Volume 195: Persistent Sadness
Volume 196: Obesity, Food Addiction
Volume 197: Parents of Abused Children
Volume 198: Letting Go and Letting Be
Volume 199: Childhood Sexual Abuse
Volume 200: Fear of Loss

www.ingramcontent.com/pod-product-compliance
Lightning Source LLC
Chambersburg PA
CBHW030501220526
45464CB00006B/2606